Extraordinary!

A Book for Children with Rare Diseases

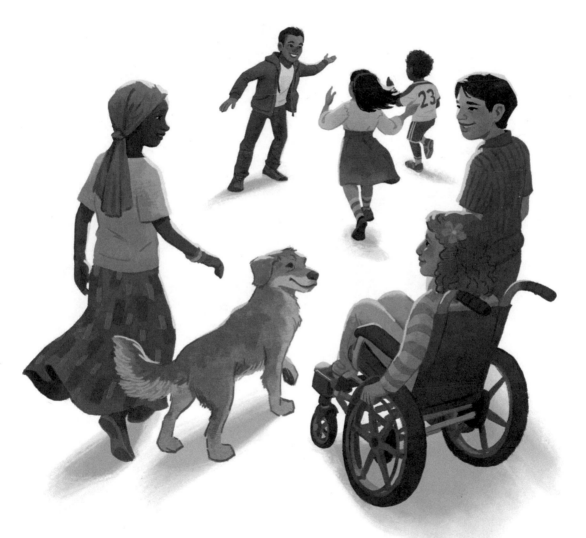

By **Evren** and **Kara Ayik**

Illustrated by **Ian Dale**

This book is dedicated to all children

around the world who have a rare disease and

in memory of those children with rare diseases

who have finished their earthly journey.

We are a family.

EXTRAORDINARY!
A Book for Children with Rare Diseases
Published by Kara A. Ayik

www.rarediseasebookforkids.com

Text © 2021 Evren & Kara Ayik
Illustrations © 2021 Ian Dale

Library of Congress Control Number: 2020925835
ISBN (Paperback): 978-1-7360344-0-8
ISBN (Hardcover): 978-1-7360344-8-4
eISBN: 978-1-7360344-9-1

First Edition 2021

Hi! My name is Evren, and my mom and I have written this book for you.

You and I are very special people. There is no one else in the world exactly like you or me. Even if someone has the same name as you or looks just like you, no one is exactly the same as you. Each human being in the world has a unique *identity*.

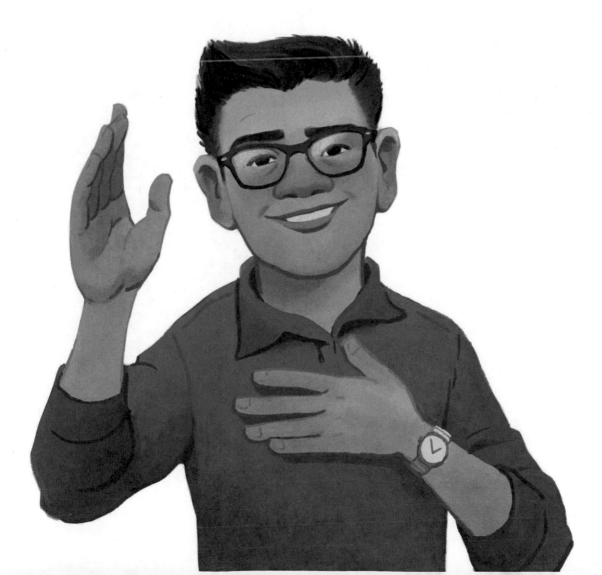

An identity is what makes *me* who I am and what makes *you* who you are. Identities are made of many pieces, just like a puzzle. A puzzle is made of many different pieces all connected together to create a wonderful picture.

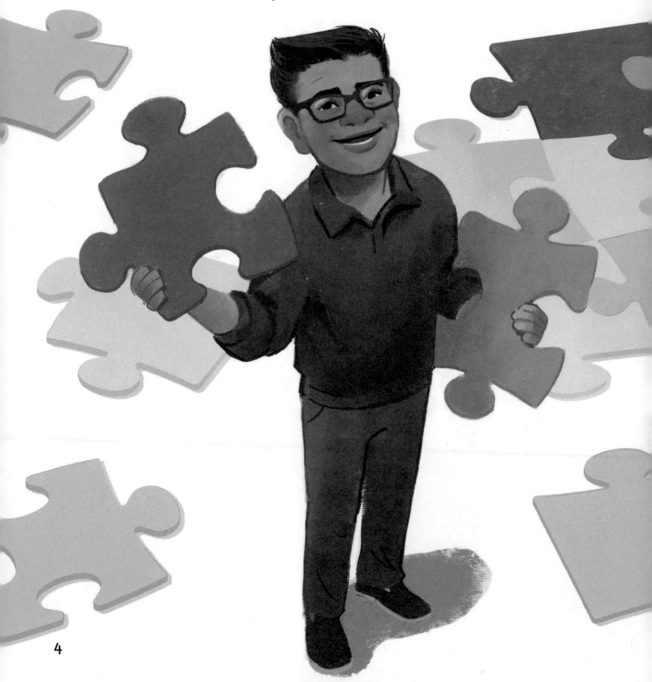

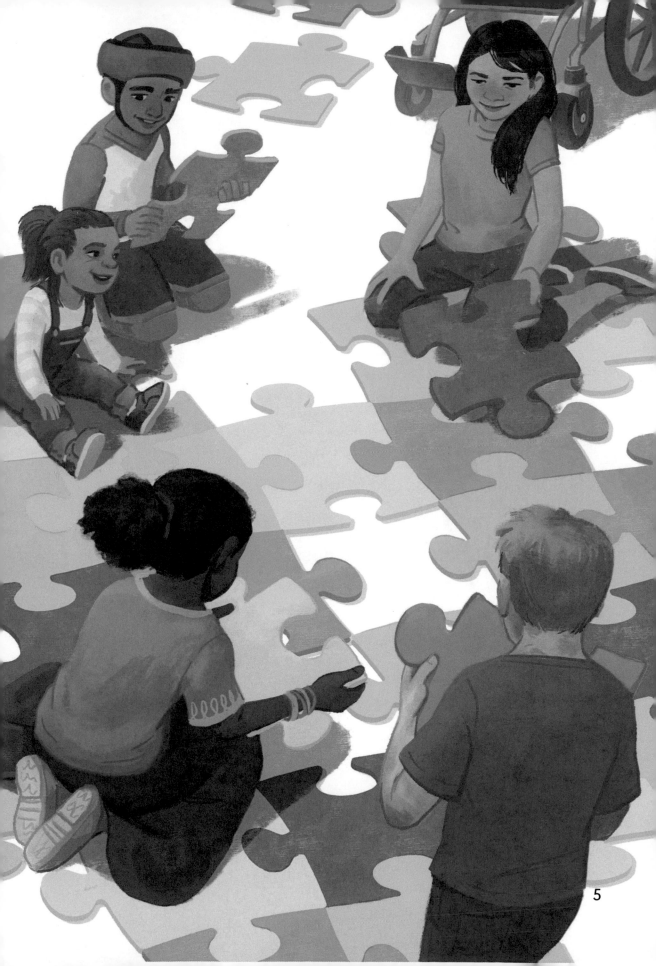

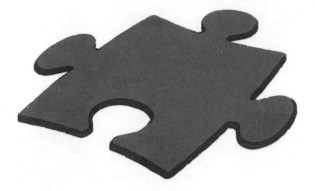

One piece of our identity is our *personality*.

Are you quiet and cheerful like me? Or are you noisy and active? Do you like to read books or collect stickers? Do you enjoy sports, doing art projects, or listening to music?

What we like and how we express ourselves are parts of our personality. Just like another puzzle, our personality is also made of distinct pieces, and these pieces are called *traits*. Being funny or shy or active are examples of personality traits.

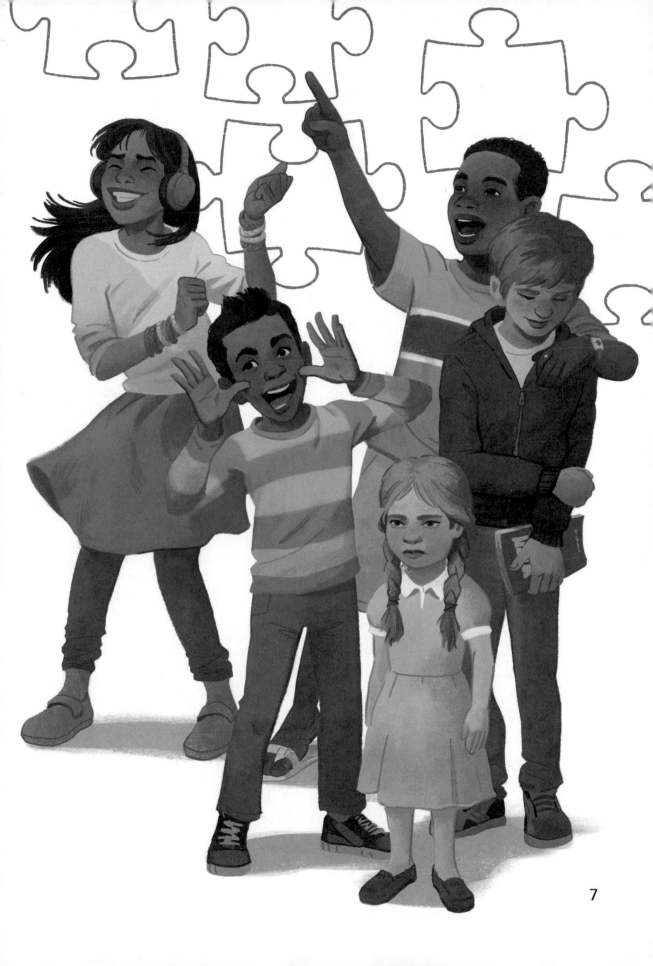

More pieces of our identity include our talents or abilities, which I call *gifts*. Sometimes we don't know what our gifts are, but everyone has them, and so do you. It may take time to discover what your gifts are, although you may already know some of them.

Are you an artist or singer? Do animals or small children seem to really like you? Are you an excellent student? One of my gifts is that I have a great imagination, and people tell me I have a big heart!

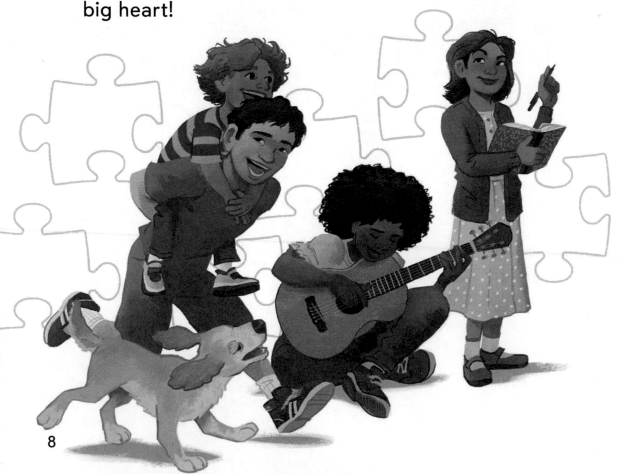

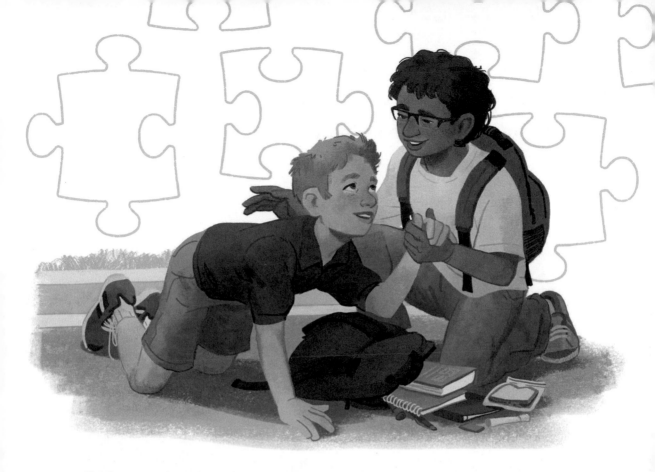

Other pieces of our identity are our *character qualities*. Character qualities are the voices of our hearts and minds that make us think, behave, or act the ways we do. Sometimes we are born with character qualities, but we can also learn them from our families, our teachers, or our experiences.

Three of my character qualities are patience, kindness, and honesty. These qualities help me to make decisions about what I say and do, like always offering to help others and never taking anything that doesn't belong to me.

The way we look on the outside is part of our identity. No one else in the world looks exactly like you do. Even if you have an identical twin, there will be small differences in your *appearance*.

My hair is dark brown, and my eyes are hazel. My eyelashes and eyebrows are thick and dark. What do you look like? Do you have red hair or black hair? Maybe your eyes are brown? Or blue?

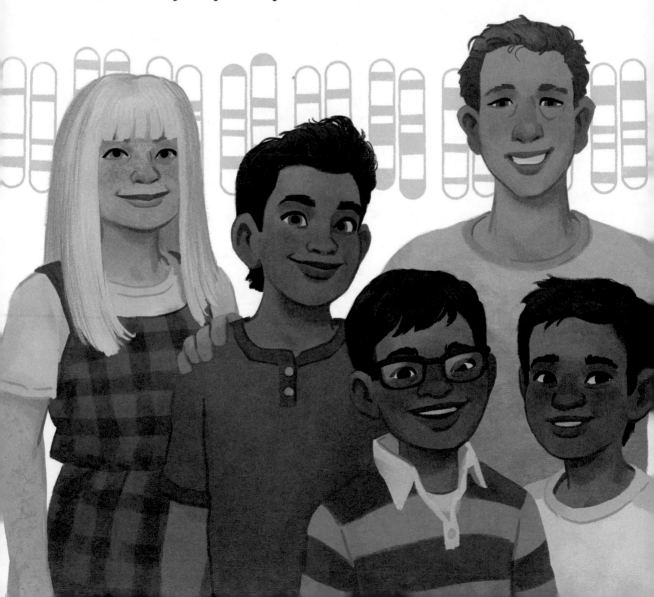

Have you ever wondered why we all look different?

Our genes, or the instructions that tell our bodies much of what we should look like and how our bodies should work, are all different as well. Did you know that no one else in the world has the same fingerprints as you do? That is because of our genes and our bodies' development that begins before we are born.

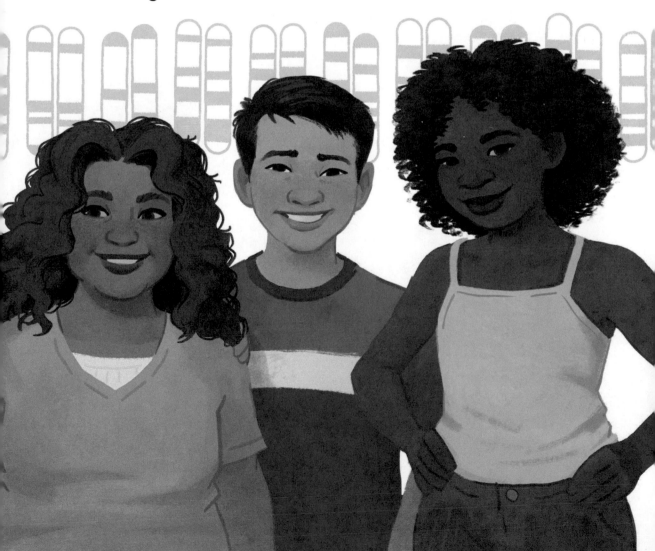

Sometimes, our genes change the instructions our human bodies usually follow, and that is why some of us have a rare disease. A rare disease is one that very few people in the world have. There are many different diseases that are considered rare. My rare disease is called ASMD, and having ASMD makes it hard for my body to break down a certain type of fat.

What is your rare disease? Can you pronounce it correctly and explain it using simple words?

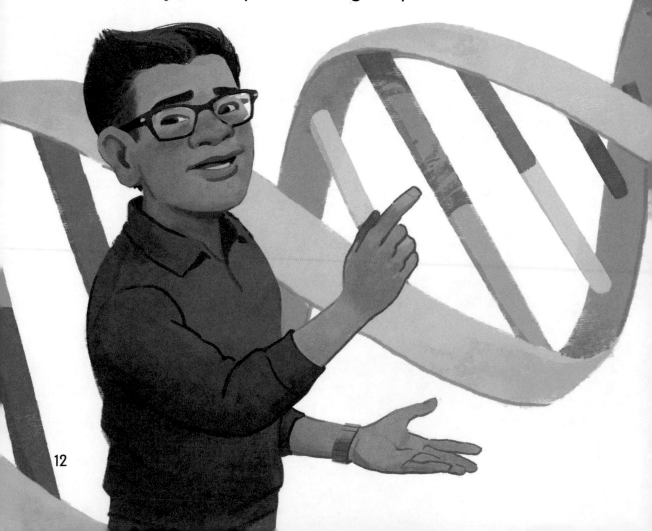

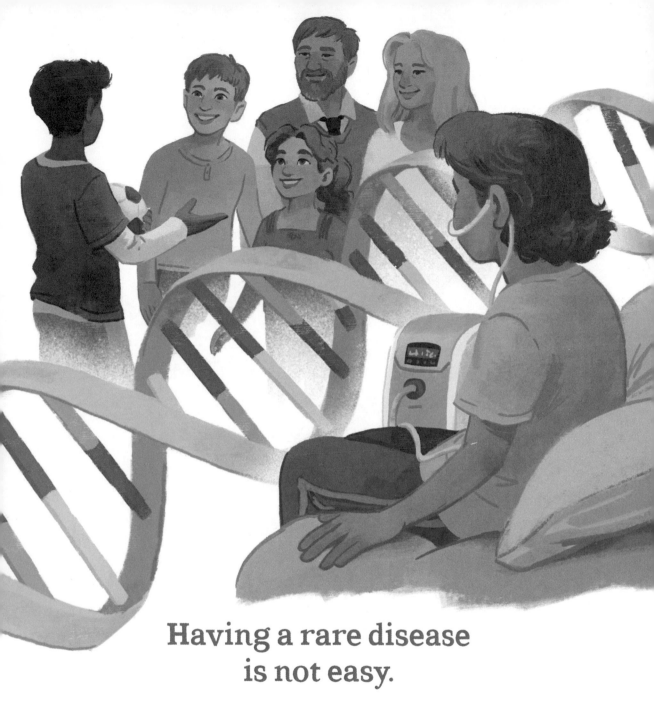

Having a rare disease is not easy.

Sometimes, no one else in our family shares our rare disease, and no one else we know has our rare disease. That can be lonely. You may feel as though no one in the world really understands what life is like for you.

Sometimes, our rare diseases make our bodies work differently, so we need tools that help our bodies work better like glasses, hearing aids, walkers, oxygen (air for breathing), or wheelchairs.

We might also need to take different kinds of medicines like liquids or pills, injections, and infusions. Some children will spend time in the hospital.

When I was growing up, I needed glasses, medicines like pills and vitamins, and physical therapy to make my arms and legs more flexible. Often I had to go to the doctor for appointments and medical tests. I really did not like that at all. I did not want to miss school, and I did not like to be poked with needles when I needed a blood test.

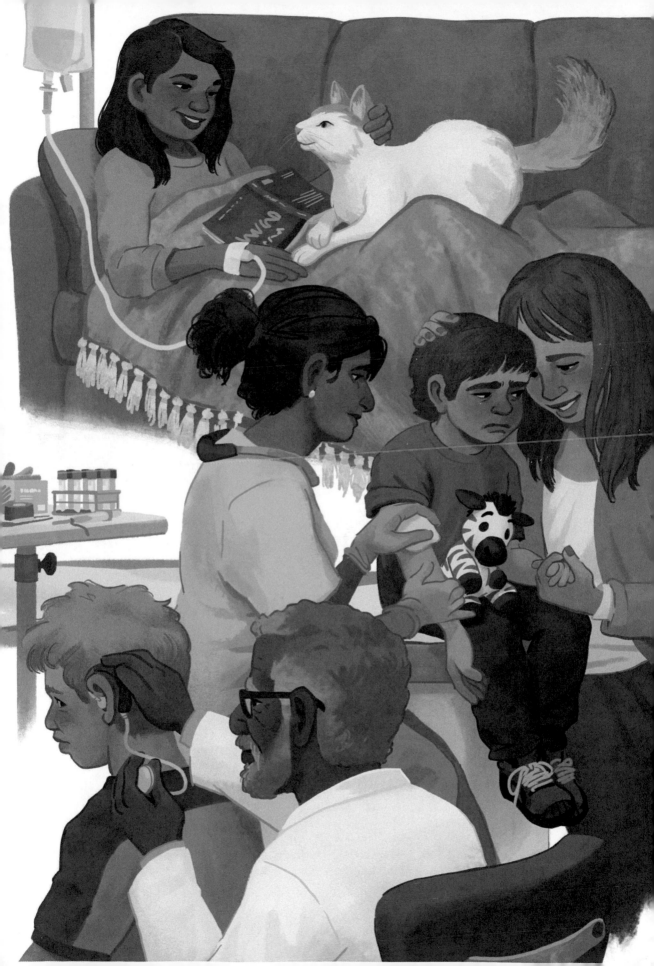

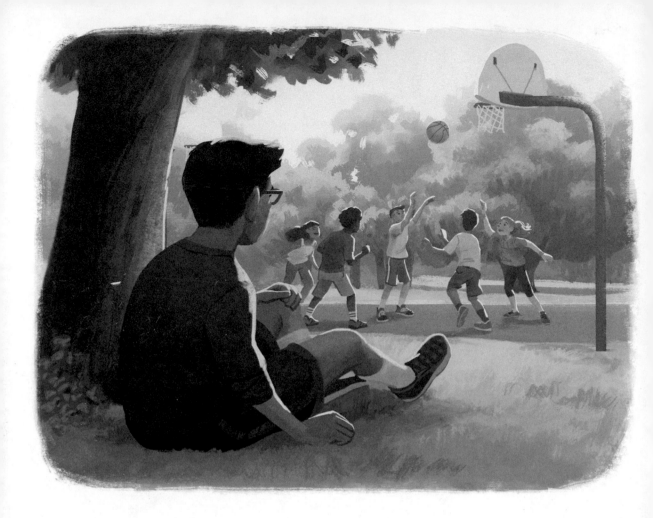

Needing these tools, tests, and clinic visits can be frustrating. At times we may wish we did not need anything to make our bodies work better. We may wish we were just like other children who do not have a rare disease, maybe even like our own brothers or sisters. At times I felt jealous of my brother who does not have a rare disease. He could play sports and make friends easily. Have you ever felt jealous of someone like I did, or wished you did not have a rare disease?

When people see or hear about how our rare diseases affect us, like the ways our faces or bodies are different, or the medicine or tools we need, they react in different ways. They may be curious about these effects, and they may also feel confused, troubled, or scared.

Have you ever felt curious? How about confused, troubled, or scared? The answer is probably yes. Human beings all have these feelings at times. We may feel that way when we encounter something new that we cannot fully understand or accept right away.

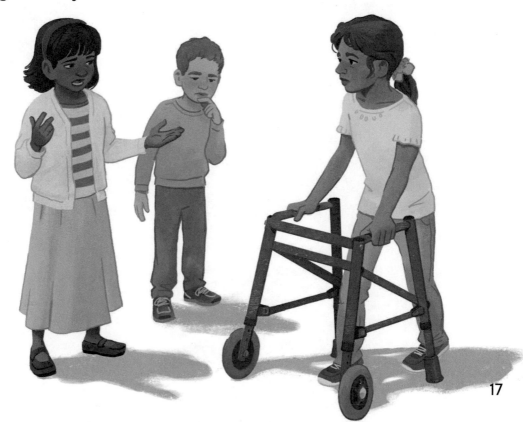

When children, teenagers, or even grownups feel curious, confused, troubled, or scared, they may express their thoughts or feelings in ways that may hurt our feelings. They may accidentally say words or behave in ways that make us feel bad. Sometimes, people are unkind because it makes them feel powerful. If that happens, the most important thing to remember is that they cannot yet see and understand the value of your unique and magnificent identity.

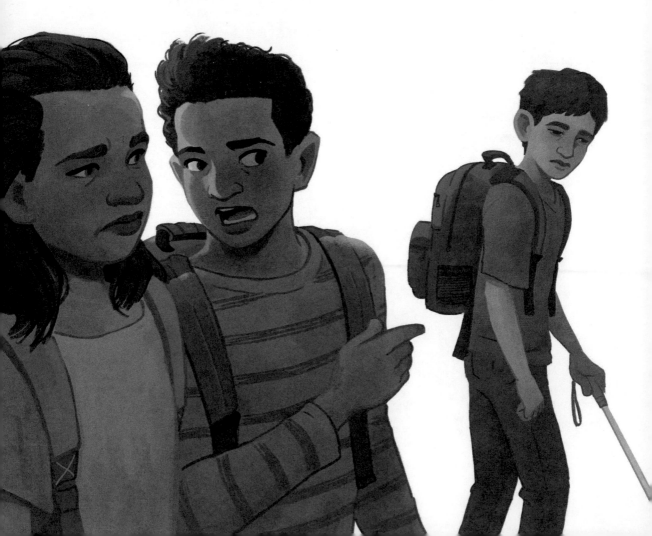

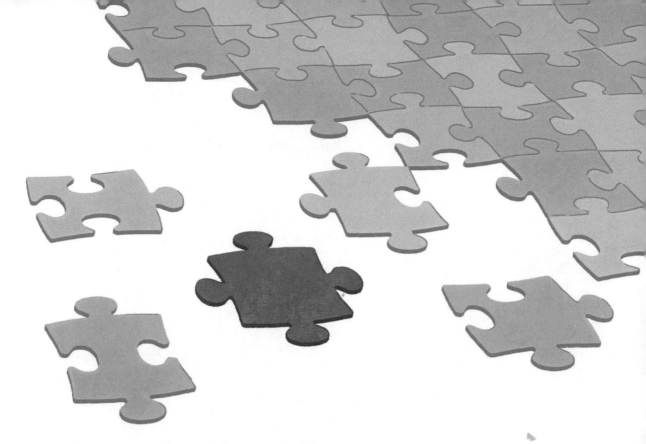

Some people do not realize that our identities are made up of many different pieces, and that they will never meet someone else exactly like you or me. Human beings notice and pay attention to things that are different, and because of that, they may focus on only one single piece of our identity, like our rare disease. That's just like looking at one single puzzle piece instead of the entire puzzle put together.

You might choose to help people discover the other pieces of your identity, like the activities you enjoy or the gifts you have.

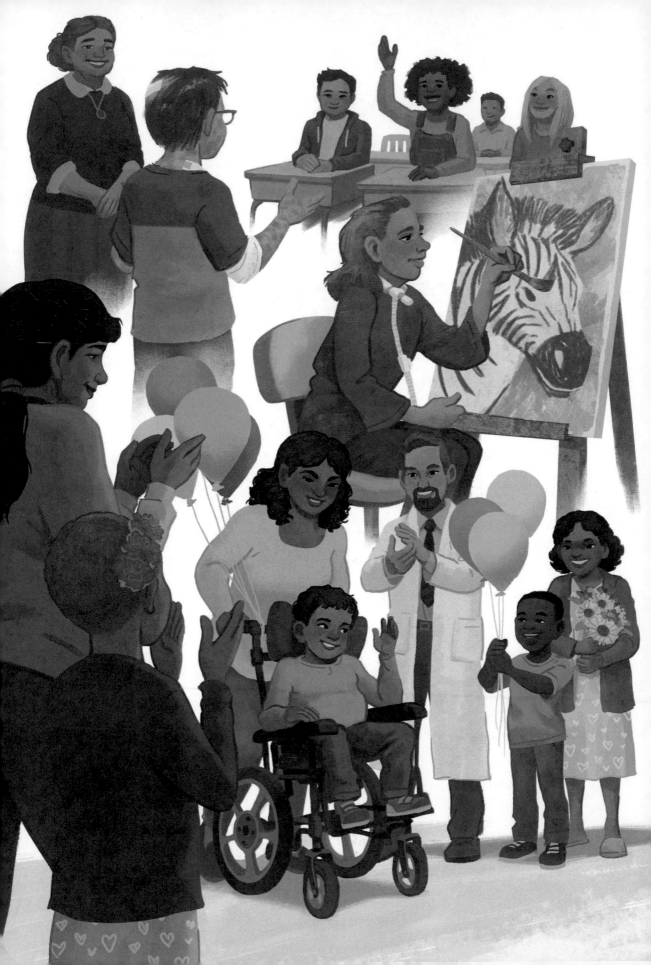

You may be surprised to hear this, but did you know that anyone with a rare disease—even a kid—can be a teacher? Because having a rare disease allows us to see and experience life in ways that others can't, we become the ones who teach kids and adults all kinds of lessons about being a human being.

For example, we can teach them about what it means to be brave, patient, and strong. We can teach them lessons about the human body and how our bodies work differently. Best of all, you and I have the power to inspire people and make them laugh or feel joy!

Did you know that having a rare disease can allow us to discover and grow our gifts and character qualities in fantastic ways? I learned that I could speak to big groups of adults when I began sharing stories about my life with a rare disease.

And, I think that even though I was born with a kind personality, having a rare disease has taught me a lot about compassion, or caring about other people's needs and feelings. Enduring all the medical appointments and tests made me braver and stronger.

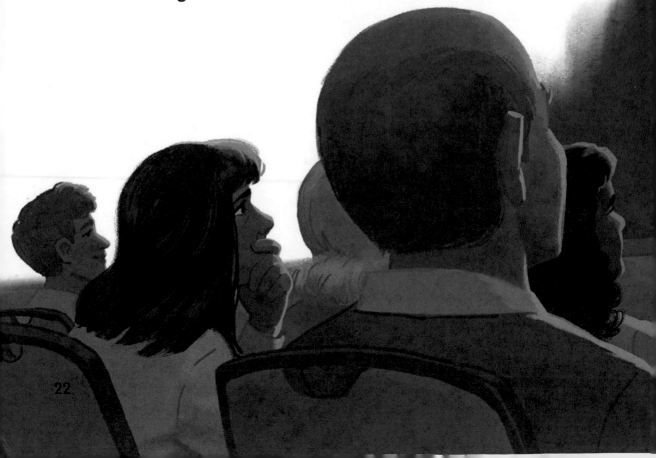

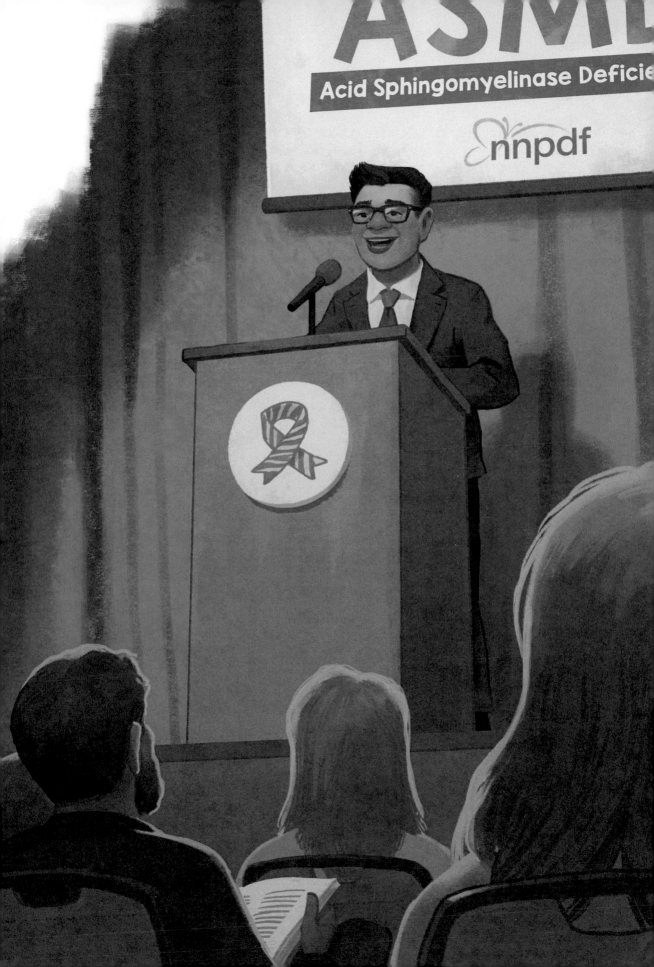

Yes, I did feel lonely at times when I was growing up because of my rare disease, but as I grew older, I learned that there are other children and grown-ups in the world who also have my same rare disease.

I met a few of them in person, and some of them I met over the internet. If you and your family begin searching on the internet, you will probably find an organization that will help you meet other kids with your rare disease.

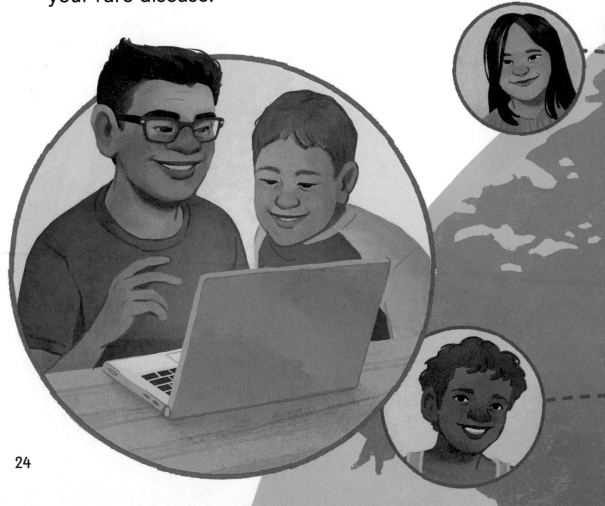

Or, you may meet kids who have a rare disease that is different from your own, but who still understand your thoughts and feelings. Your new friends may live in different countries around the world. That's exciting!

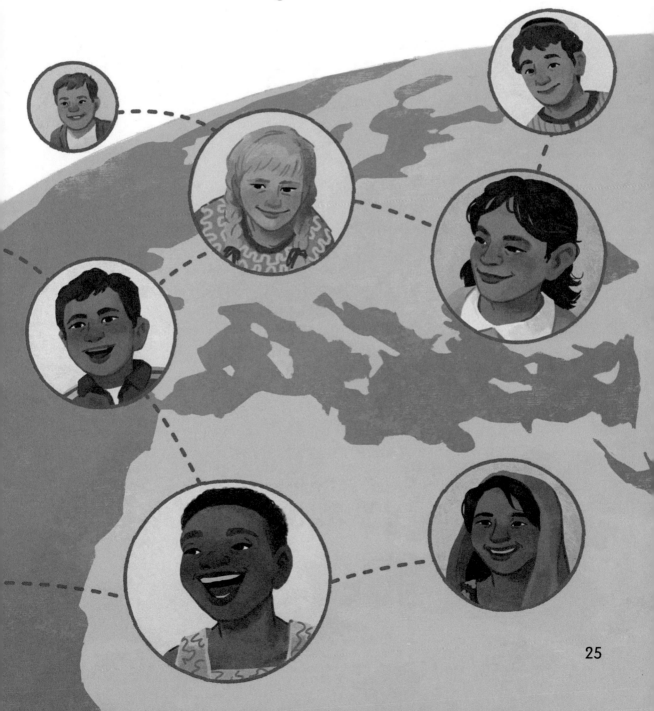

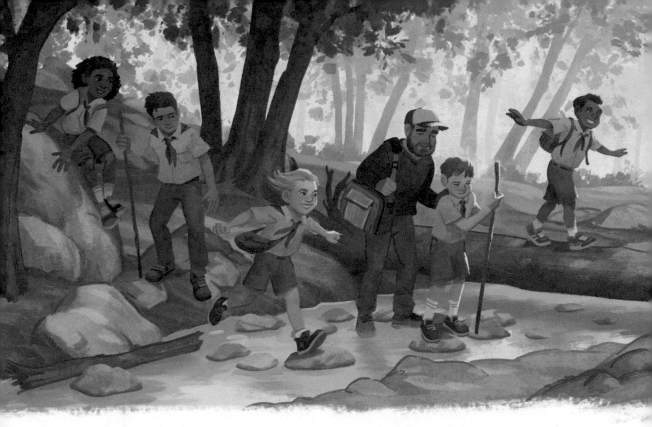

When I became a teenager, I realized that there were other children and teenagers who also had some noticeable differences about their identities, even though they did not have a rare disease. I also discovered that some kids and grown-ups are more accepting of differences.

I made new friends by joining clubs and sharing my gifts where they were needed. Eventually, I did not feel as lonely as before. **Remember that all human beings feel lonely at times, even when they do not have a rare disease.**

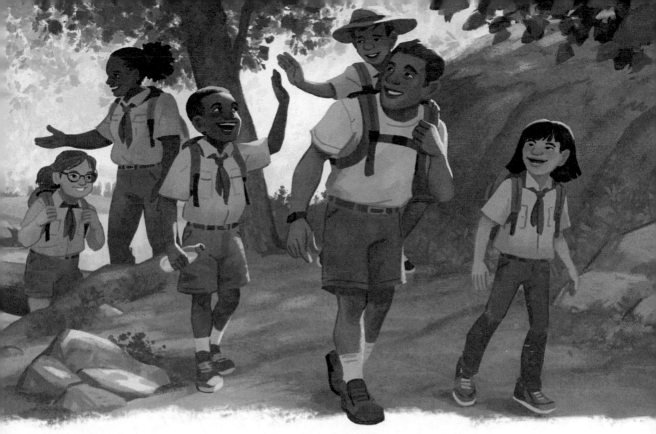

Something I want you to think about is having _fun_! Just because you have a rare disease does not mean you have to spend a lot of your time and energy thinking about it. Also, you don't have to just watch other kids do fun activities. With some thinking and courage, you and your grown-ups can find ways for you to join in.

I like treasure hunting, camping, skateboarding, and watching football games. How about you? You probably already have activities you enjoy, and you will discover even more if you seek out new adventures.

What is most important to remember from our book is that you are a very special person because of your unique identity! And, you are not special just because you have a rare disease. Millions of people in the world have some kind of rare disease.

You are special because you have your own one-of-a-kind identity that is made up of many pieces, and having a rare disease is just one of them.

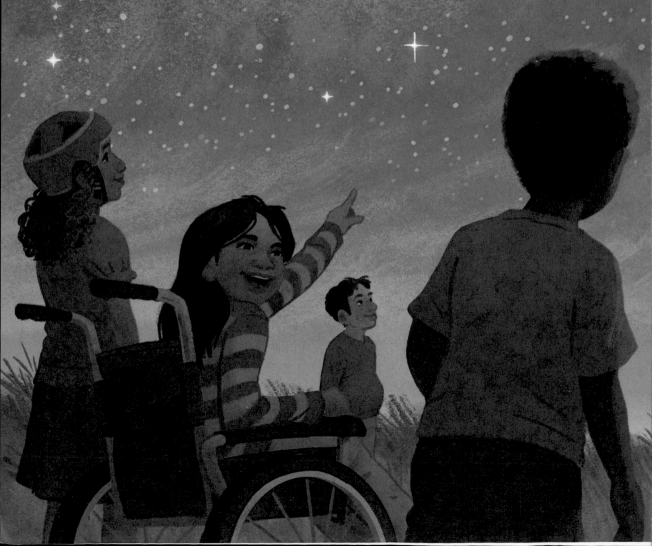

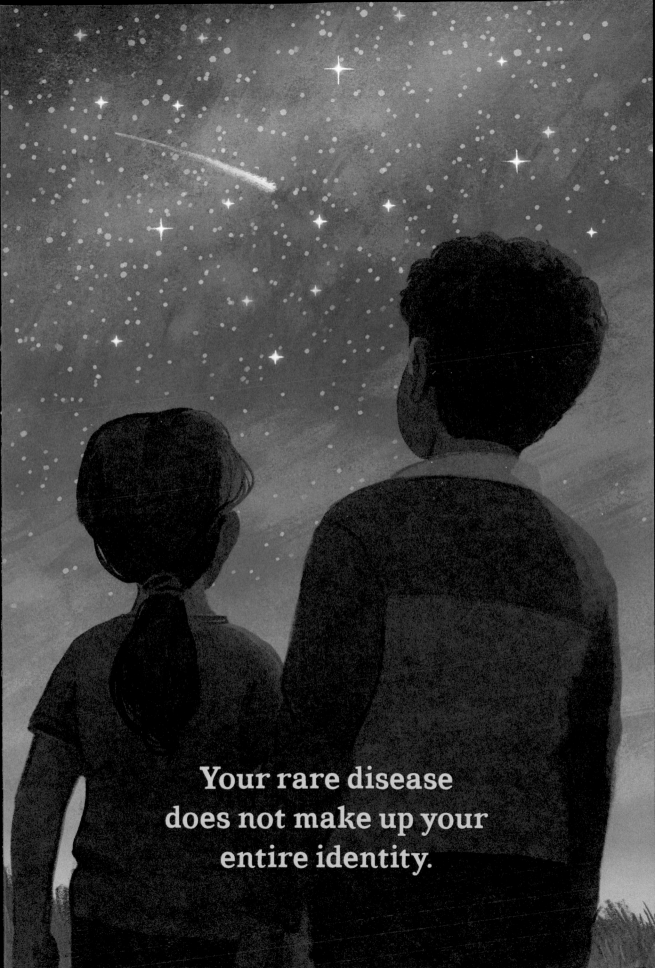

Your rare disease
does not make up your
entire identity.

Living with a rare disease may not be easy, but if we persevere, or never give up, we will grow so much from all the lessons our rare disease can help us learn.

We have a unique purpose in this world, and our rare diseases can play an important part of helping us to become the EXTRAORDINARY individuals we are intended to be.

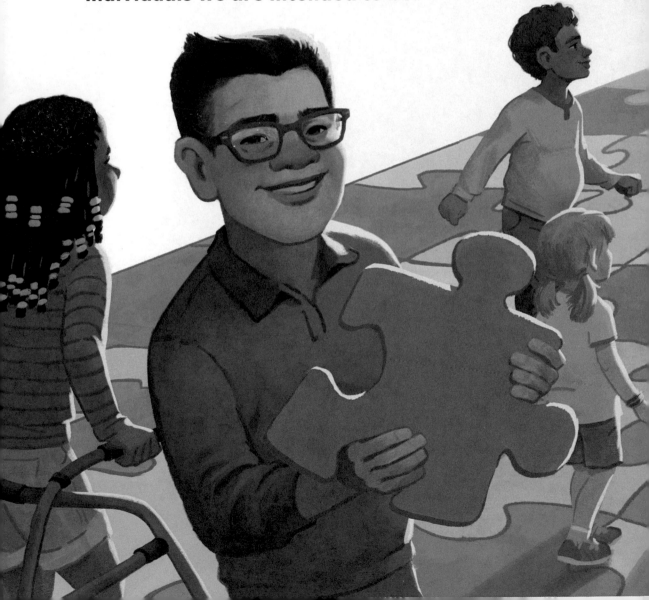

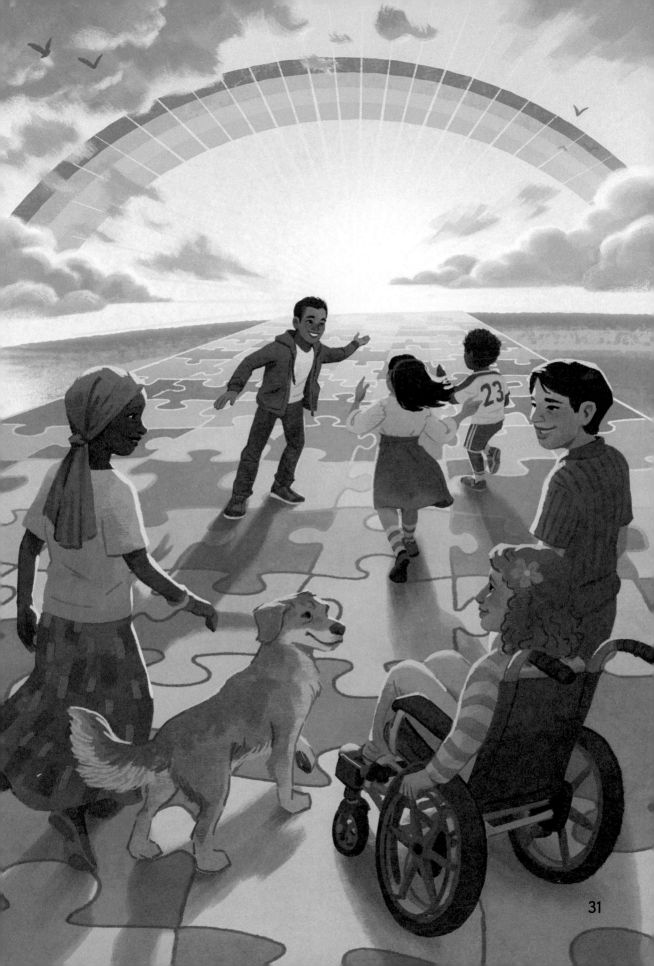

About the Creators

Evren & Kara Ayik wrote this book to uplift children with rare diseases following Evren's graduation from high school.

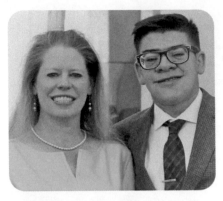

Evren's advocacy work for people with ASMD began in 2017 when he was invited to speak at the FDA in Maryland. He went on to speak to audiences in several other states about life with ASMD to raise awareness of and support for treatments for rare diseases. In 2019, he earned the rank of Eagle Scout and was a California Boy's State delegate in Sacramento. Evren is also the winner of the prestigious TORCH Award for rare disease advocacy from Sanofi Genzyme. He plans to become a special education teacher and now attends California State University, Fresno.

His mother, Kara, has been an educator for over twenty years and believes that children must cultivate true self-worth and values to help them navigate their journeys through life. Her greatest joy and proudest accomplishment has been raising her two sons, Evren and Erol. Above all, Evren and Kara seek to promote compassion and respect for children with rare diseases and special needs.

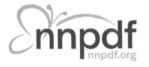
nnpdf.org

Learn more about ASMD by visiting the National Niemann Pick Disease Foundation's website at www.nndpdf.org

Ian Dale explores how visual art can amplify the stories of those less visible among us. He frequently illustrates for non-profit and faith-based organizations and publishers, and his work has been available to kids around the world. Ian lives in Southern California with his wife and two young children. See more of his work online at www.iandale.net.

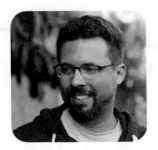